MANUAL HANDLING
An Ergonomic Approach

by
Dr Stephen Pheasant
Ergonomics Advisor
National Back Pain Association

and

Professor David Stubbs
Robens Institute
University of Surrey

NBPA

The National Back Pain Association

FOREWORD

Employment Secretary David Hunt recently met representatives of the NBPA with their local MP Toby Jessel.

'Manual handling injuries at work are a serious problem, accounting for over a quarter of all injuries reported to the Health and Safety Executive (HSE). Sprains, strains and injuries - to the back, especially - account for the largest proportion of these, but there are also significant injuries to other parts of the body. This heavy toll causes considerable pain and suffering to the victims and their families and can often result in permanent disability.

Furthermore, these injuries represent considerable costs to employers from sickness, absence from work, compensation claims, reduced productivity and damages to goods; and to the country through demands on health and social services. The country's annual toll from manual handling injuries and other forms of occupational musculoskeletal disorder is estimated at between £1.25 and £1.75 billion.

These figures give me considerable cause for concern and I am very happy, therefore, to commend this edition of 'Manual Handling - An Ergonomic Approach', a book which is already well known and respected throughout industry as 'Lifting and Handling - An Ergonomic Approach'.

This new, extended, edition takes account of the EC Manual Handling Operations Regulations 1992 and the HSE's guidance on them. 'Manual Handling - An Ergonomic Approach' provides good advice on avoiding the causes of manual handling injury, on carrying out assesments and on training. I am particularly pleased to see it emphasised that the most effective way to reduce manual handling injury, and especially back injury, is through avoiding manual handling wherever possible and designing safer systems of work using the ergonomic approach.

I am sure that employers and workers in all industries will benefit from following the guidance provided by this book. By doing so workers will safeguard their health, and employers will have a healthier and more effective workforce.

I congratulate the National Back Pain Association for addressing the problem by offering such a readable solution and valuable teaching aid.'

Rt Hon David Hunt MBE MP
Secretary of State for Employment

THE NATIONAL BACK PAIN ASSOCIATION

Founded in 1968, the National Back Pain Association is the only organisation which focuses all its efforts on back pain.

Supported entirely by voluntary donations, the NBPA's mission is:

- to fund patient-oriented scientific research into the causes and treatment of back pain;

- to educate people in sensible use of the body, thereby reducing the incidence of back pain, and;

- to help form and support self-help branches through which back pain sufferers and those who care for them may receive information, advice and mutual help.

First published 1991 as 'Lifting and Handling: An Ergonomic Approach'
This edition 1994

Published by The National Back Pain Association, 16 Elmtree Road, Teddington, Middlesex TW11 8ST. Telephone: 081-977 5474.

Original design by Redesign. This edition designed and printed by Graphic Impressions, 13-14 Great Sutton Street, London EC1 Telephone: 071-253 5444.

A catalogue record for this publication is available from the British Library.

ISBN 0 9507726 8 2

CONTENTS

CONTENTS

ACKNOWLEDGEMENTS

The lifting procedures described in the section of the present work which deal with 'training' are based extensively upon those described in an earlier NBPA publication entitled 'Lifting Instructors' Manual'. The authors of the present work would like to acknowledge the contribution made by the authors of the earlier work; C.R. Hayne and J.D.G. Troup, and illustrator Don Charlesworth.

The NBPA wishes to thank Thorn EMI for their support in financing this publication.

DISCLAIMER

The risks associated with manual handling tasks are complex – and to some extent they are unpredictable. In preparing this text every reasonable attempt has been made to ensure that the advice which is given conforms to what would currently be regarded as 'good working practice'. The reader is warned, however, that there are no infallible rules in this area and each situation must be judged on its own merits. Neither the authors nor the publishers can accept responsibility for any consequences which might result from decisions made upon the basis of the advice given herein.

BACK PAIN AT WORK

INTRODUCTION

Back pain is an extremely common condition. Four out of every five adults in this country will suffer from one or more episodes of back pain during the course of their lives. At any point in time, about one person in seven will be suffering from back pain.

Recent figures show that 14 per cent of all certified sickness absence in the UK is due to back pain. The figure is climbing steadily. The annual cost of this sickness absence is thought to be in the order of £5000 million.

Most attacks of back pain clear up within a few weeks – although a small minority of cases may lead to prolonged periods of disability. Back pain tends to be recurrent; that is, once you have had one attack you are very much more likely to have others. About 50% of people who have time off work because of back problems have another attack within a year; and the likelihood of a recurrence increases with the number of attacks that an individual has.

Some people with long-standing back trouble have repeated attacks of pain, separated by relatively long periods during which their backs seem to be more or less normal. During these pain-free periods they can do quite heavy work without discomfort. Other people find that they have a dull ache in their back almost all of the time. The discomfort is aggravated by certain characteristic activities and at times it will flare up into episodes of intense pain.

Back pain is equally common in men and women, and it occurs at all ages; but it is particularly common in people whose work involves certain types of activity. We call these activities **risk factors**. In people who are not exposed to these risks, back pain is really quite rare. A person's work may not be the sole cause of his back pain; but it is likely to be a significant contributory factor in very many cases. If nothing is done about those aspects of an individual's working life which cause his back problems, we should not be surprised if these problems are recurrent.

Back pain has been the subject of a great deal of research and although there is much that we still do not know about the subject, the sorts of working activities which are likely to place people at risk are reasonably well known.

Back pain has been found to be associated with:

- **heavy manual work – lifting and handling, forceful exertion, bending, twisting etc**

- **working in a stooped position**

- **prolonged sitting in a fixed position**

- **vibration**

- **psychological stress**

This publication is mainly concerned with manual handling. But it is important to realise that the effects of the various activities which lead to back trouble, are likely to be cumulative. The work of a delivery driver, for example, may involve prolonged sitting in a fixed position, with vibration exposure as well as heavy lifting. Similarly, the work of a nurse may require her to spend long periods of time in a stooped position and may be psychologically stressful, as well as being physically very demanding.

Are some sorts of people more at risk than others, given that they are doing the same kind of work? Since back pain is commonly recurrent, it follows that a person with a history of the condition is likely to be at a higher level of risk. The magnitude of this risk will depend on the extent to which the previous episodes of the condition have left the back vulnerable to further injury; but in practice this may be difficult to determine. Some studies have shown that tall people may be more prone to back trouble than short people, but there is really very little in it. Some people may be at risk because of the anatomical make-up of their spines, but except for certain relatively rare conditions, the effects are again small.

Strength and fitness are very much more important. In general, the stronger and fitter you are, the less likely you are to injure your back doing heavy work. Smokers are also more susceptible to back trouble than non-smokers, although we do not really know why. Statistically speaking, your chances of having serious back problems increase by about 20% for every ten cigarettes per day that you smoke. So this is yet another very good reason for giving it up.

Sometimes an attack of back pain comes on suddenly and the individual concerned regards it (rightly or wrongly) as having been caused by the activity they were engaged in at the time. But equally often the condition has an insidious onset and the victim is unable to attribute it to any activity in particular (see Fig. 1).

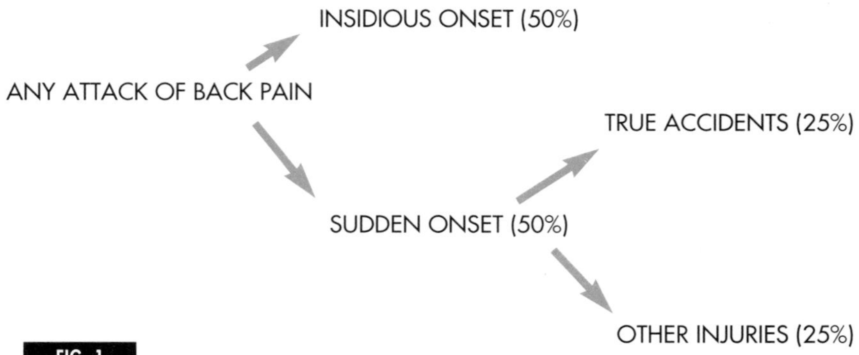

INSIDIOUS ONSET (50%)

ANY ATTACK OF BACK PAIN

TRUE ACCIDENTS (25%)

SUDDEN ONSET (50%)

OTHER INJURIES (25%)

FIG. 1

The episodes of sudden onset may be divided, more or less equally, into two further categories. About half are true accidents such as slips and falls; situations where a load gets out of hand and so on. The other half are not really accidents in the strict sense of the word, although they will often be classed as such for administrative purposes, and in practical terms it is perfectly reasonable that they should. In these cases, the back injury occurs during the course of a normal working activity, performed in what seems to be the ordinary way. Lifting injuries may fall into either category. Some manual handling injuries, which do not involve true accidents, are obviously attributable to overexertion: the individual overstrains himself trying to shift a load which is beyond his capacity or handling a more modest load in an awkward position. It is also quite common for an attack of back pain to come on as an individual straightens up after a period in a stooped position, whether or not he is handling a load at the time.

The fact that an episode of back pain came on gradually, rather than during the course of a specific working activity, does not mean that the person's work was not its principal cause. Heavy lifting may result in cumulative damage to the spine over a period of time, leading to an insidious onset of symptoms. That an episode of back pain comes on suddenly, as the individual attempts a particular lifting action, does not mean that it was caused by that particular action alone. The cumulative effects of heavy lifting may leave a person's back in a vulnerable state in which it is susceptible to injury; the point at which the 'injury' occurs may be more or less a matter of chance.

About one quarter of all certified accidents at work are due to manual handling activities. Of these approximately half are back injuries. The remainder involve the hands, feet, arms, legs etc. The sorts of activities relating to these back injuries are very varied and encompass lifting, lowering, holding, carrying, pushing, pulling and throwing. In most types of industrial work, the load will be an inert object, but in other contexts it could be a human being [1] or an animal. In a few cases, the 'load' is an immovable object, like a machine part that is stuck in place or an excessively stiff lever or control.

In seeking to establish safe working practices with regard to manual tasks, it is necessary to consider three principal kinds of risks:

- **the risk of overexertion**
  Due to a load which is beyond the capacity of the individual concerned, given the circumstances under which she is required to lift it

- **the risk of cumulative damage**
  Due to repetitive lifting, fixed working posture and so on

- **the risk of accidental injury**
  In practice, these risks very frequently occur in combination and it may be difficult to separate them in any particular case

In theory there are three possible ways of dealing with these risks:

- selection

- training

- ergonomics

The extent to which the selection of workers is a viable option will depend, in part, upon the state of the labour market. But even where recruitment presents little or no problem, it is still genuinely difficult to determine which individuals are likely to be most at risk in a given situation. Where possible, it obviously makes sense to allocate the heaviest jobs to the biggest and strongest people; and to transfer people

---

[1] For detailed advice on lifting people, read 'The Guide to the Handling of Patients', also published by the NBPA.

who are known to be unfit to lighter forms of work. Beyond these fairly simple commonsense precautions, the scope for more sophisticated selection procedures is likely to be limited.

Training has been the most popular approach to dealing with these problems in the past. Training programmes of the conventional kind tend to be based on the assumption that back injuries generally result from faulty lifting technique. There is little real evidence for this belief; and although most people who run training programmes have their own favourite success stories which they like to tell, the evidence available at the present time suggests that successful training programmes are the exception rather than the rule.

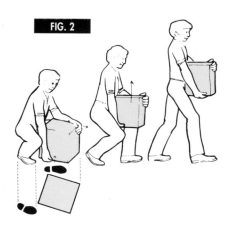

FIG. 2

There are a number of reasons why this might be the case. It is perfectly true that lifting is generally an unconsidered, unplanned kind of action. We do it automatically, without thinking. It is also true that there are often good ways and bad ways of lifting a particular load; or at the least, some ways which are less hazardous than others. The real trouble often comes in situations where the nature of the load or the design of the working environment prevents the individual from lifting in a safe way, however well trained he may be.

Fig. 2 illustrates what is generally considered to be a good lifting technique. Details of this lift will be examined later. The problem is that it can only be done this way if there is a compact load, an unobstructed work area, and the load is to be lifted within a limited range of heights.

It follows, therefore, that lifting training can only be effective in the context of an overall strategy for designing safe systems of work – or to be more precise, **safer** systems of work, because the total elimination of risk is generally an unattainable ideal. This is what is meant by the 'ergonomic approach'.

THE EC DIRECTIVE AND HSE GUIDANCE

In May 1990 the Council of the European Community published a Directive on:

'The minimum health and safety requirements for the handling of loads where there is a risk, particularly of back injury, to workers'.

Each European member state is now required to implement this Directive. The statutory body responsible for so doing in the UK is the Health and Safety Commission (HSC).

In response to the Directive, the HSE (Health and Safety Executive) has outlined a clear hierarchy of measures. In essence, the employer will be required to:

- **avoid hazardous manual handling operations so far as is reasonably practicable;**

- **assess any hazardous handling operations that cannot be avoided, and;**

- **reduce the risk of injury so far as is reasonably practicable using assessment as a basis for action.**

SAFE SYSTEMS OF WORK

The first stage of any effective programme for preventing manual handling injuries is a thorough investigation of current working practices. This will generally necessitate both direct observation and discussions with the people involved. It is important to find out about the unofficial short cuts that people take as well as the 'official' way of doing things. Foremen and supervisors sometimes turn a blind eye to these practices in order to get the job done on time. Accident records and sickness absence figures may help to pinpoint areas of high risk.

Accounts of 'near misses', where an accident was narrowly avoided, are another important source of data.

In terms of back pain prevention, the overall objective of this investigation will be to determine those aspects of the working situation which are likely to lead to an unreasonably high level of loading on the person's back. It is necessary to take into account:

- **dynamic loading** due to lifting and handling actions and other vigorous physical activity

- **static loading** due to holding actions, stooped postures and so on

Having identified the most important sources of loading, a coherent plan for dealing with the problem can be made. Some sources of loading can be eliminated by training people to work in a different way. However, many will require changes in the design of the working system. To recognise these options, we need to first understand some basic principles of anatomy and body mechanics.

BODY MECHANICS

ANATOMY

The human spine is a flexible column of 24 bones called vertebrae, plus a larger wedge shaped bone at the bottom, which is called the sacrum (Fig. 3). The uppermost vertebra supports the skull and the sacrum articulates with the hip bones at the sacroiliac joints. There are seven cervical vertebrae in the neck. The ribs are attached in pairs to each of the twelve thoracic vertebrae and there are five lumbar vertebrae in the small of the back. Some people actually have four or six lumbar vertebrae, but it does not seem to affect them in any way.

In discussing anatomy and lifting, the lumbar region (Fig. 4) is the most important area. Although any part of the spine or trunk may be damaged during manual handling activities, it is the lumbar spine and its adjacent structures that tend to be damaged most frequently.

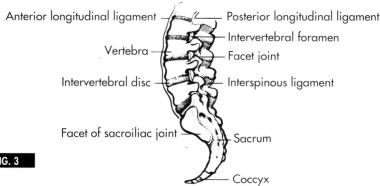

Anterior longitudinal ligament — Posterior longitudinal ligament
Intervertebral foramen
Vertebra — Facet joint
Intervertebral disc — Interspinous ligament

Facet of sacroiliac joint — Sacrum

Coccyx

FIG. 3

Between each pair of vertebrae, both in the lumbar region and elsewhere, is a tough pad of tissue called the intervertebral disc, which acts as a shock absorber. The disc has a fibrous outer layer and a fluid-filled centre. The fibres of the outer layer are arranged something like the cords of a cross-ply car tyre.

Although there is a certain amount of disagreement on the subject, most medical people now believe that only a relatively small minority of back injuries (probably not more than 5%) involve damage to the intervertebral discs. However, when they do occur, disc injuries tend to be among the more serious sorts of back problems.

Fractures of the bones of the spine are also quite rare, and almost never occur as a result of lifting actions, except when the bones have been weakened by osteoporosis – for example, in elderly women. The majority of back injuries of the ordinary kind probably involve damage to the muscles and soft tissues which support the spine and control its movements. There may also be a misalignment of the small apophyseal facet joints which lie behind the discs and such problems as the entrapment of nerve roots.

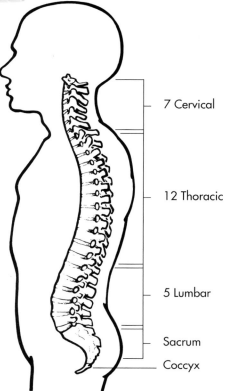

FIG. 4

7 Cervical

12 Thoracic

5 Lumbar

Sacrum

Coccyx

THE LIFTING ACTION

Fig. 5 shows a man lifting a weight in a stooped position, in which his trunk is more or less horizontal. A very simple mechanical calculation, based upon the principle of levers, demonstrates the risk involved in this action. The combined weight (W) of the load and the trunk acts at a distance (x) from the fulcrum of the lumbar spine. (The fulcrum of a lever is the point at which it pivots.) This load must be counterbalanced by a force (F) exerted by the back muscles, which act at a very much shorter distance (d) from the fulcrum. By the principle of levers:

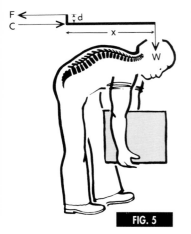

FIG. 5

$$Wx = Fd$$

In practice, this means that the tension in the muscles when lifting a load in this position can be as much as ten times greater than the weight of the load. The long muscles which run down the back have a line of pull which is near enough parallel to the spine, so any tension in these muscles results in an equal and opposite compression (C) on the spine itself. The tension in the muscles, or the compression on the spine, may result in damage.

When lifting heavy weights it is instinctive to hold one's breath and tense the abdominal muscles. This natural protective mechanism puts pressure on the abdominal cavity and thus helps relieve the loading on the spine. It is rather like having a fluid-filled cushion for the spine (Fig. 6). However, there is a risk that certain regions of the muscular walls of the abdominal cavity can fail under pressure. This is why people who lift heavy weights sometimes suffer from hernias.

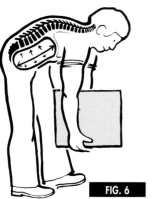

FIG. 6

Fig. 5 shows that the mechanical loading on the spine and its muscles will increase with the following three factors:

- the **weight** of the load

- the **distance** of the centre of gravity from the fulcrum of the spine

- the **inclination** of the trunk

16

Note that lifting a relatively light load held at arm's length results in the same mechanical loading on the spine and its muscles as lifting a heavier load held closer to the body. Note also that as the trunk tilts forward, its centre of gravity gets further away from the fulcrum of the spine, so the mechanical loading on the spine and its muscles increases.

Stooping to pick up even a light object from floor level may expose the spine to a considerable degree of loading by virtue of the weight of the trunk alone.

STATIC LOADING

Static muscle activities, such as holding actions and stooped postures, are more fatiguing than dynamic muscle activity of similar intensity and may result in a very much greater strain on the heart. Tasks performed with the arms in a raised position are a problem in this respect. Static loading of the intervertebral discs may lead to mechanical 'creep' effects which render them more susceptible to damage. **The elimination of static loading is therefore a high priority in the design of working systems.**

Important sources of static loading, which should be avoided wherever possible, include:

- working with the arms in a raised position

- working with the trunk in an inclined position (either forwards or to the sides)

- holding actions in which the person supports the weight of an object or holds it steady against the work piece

- struggling to lift objects which are too heavy to be moved smoothly or easily or which are stuck in place

BENDING AND TWISTING

The action of bending down to pick up an object from close to floor level has two components. The trunk as a whole tilts forward at the hips, and the spine flexes upon itself, particularly in the lumbar region (ie the back tends to become more rounded). As the lumbar spine flexes, the muscles and soft tissues come under tension and the discs are deformed. Thus the flexed spine is susceptible to damage at relatively low levels of mechanical loading.

Twisting actions are particularly hazardous, partly because of the patterns of muscle activity involved and partly because they also entail deformation of the discs. To a lesser extent this is also true for side bending actions.

The worst combination is probably a lift from floor level, involving a bending and twisting action, with the arms outstretched, after a period of working in a stooped position. Such actions are surprisingly common.

FOOT PLACEMENT

Correct foot placement is in many respects the key to safe lifting. This is partly a matter of training in correct technique, and partly a matter of the layout of the working area.

The strength of the lifting action is greatest when the line of thrust lies within the area of a person's **footbase** (represented as the shaded area in Fig. 7). Lifting strength falls off rapidly as the load moves outside this area. In part this may be due to the increased loading on the back and shoulder muscles, but it is also a matter of balance.

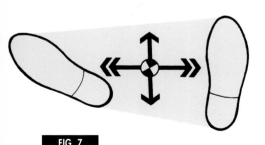

FIG. 7

When lifting a load outside the limits of the footbase, an individual has to use the weight of the body to counterbalance the weight of the load. If she slips or loses her footing, or if the load moves in an unpredictable fashion, she may suddenly find herself off balance in a way that she is unable to correct; or she may over-strain herself in trying to regain her balance.

When lifting a load outside the area of stability determined by the footbase, the individual is potentially out of balance and therefore at risk. The elimination of obstacles to optimal foot placement is therefore a high priority in the ergonomics of manual handling.

It may not always be possible to achieve this in practice. A lifting action which commences at a distance and moves into the footbase (ie towards the body), is probably preferable to one which starts in the footbase and terminates at a distance, since in the former case, the body is moving into balance and towards the area of greatest strength. But neither is desirable.

ERGONOMICS

An ergonomic assessment of a working system, in which people handle loads manually, would generally involve consideration of:

- the task – the actions performed, the overall workload, rest pauses etc.

- the load – weight, bulk, stability etc.

- the environment – work space layout, working conditions etc.

- the personnel – age, sex, strength, fitness etc.

- other factors – personal protective equipment etc.

THE WORKING AREA

In thinking about the ergonomics of manual handling tasks, it is often useful to divide up the area which surrounds the working person into vertical height ranges. It is easiest to describe these by referring to the levels of various parts of the person's body in a relaxed standing position – knee height, elbow height, shoulder height and so on. These levels will of course vary considerably between individuals, as shown in Fig. 8.

The strength of the lifting action is greatest at around knuckle height, as measured with the hands hanging by the sides. On average this is about 75 cm above the floor. The preferred height for lifting and handling tasks extends from knuckle height to elbow height or thereabouts. The zones on either side of the preferred range, from elbow height to shoulder height and from knuckle height to knee height, are somewhat less

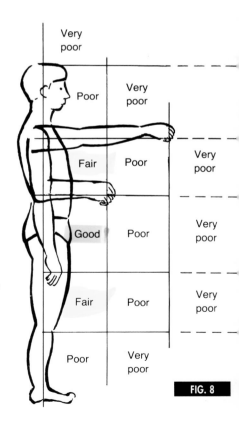

FIG. 8

satisfactory, but are acceptable provided the load is within reasonable limits. Lifting actions below knee height or above shoulder height should be avoided where possible, unless the weight of the load is low.

Lifts which commence in the lower part of the overall height range and continue into the upper part pose a particular problem. Somewhere just above elbow height a change of grip will be required. Alternatively, the lifter will have to raise his elbows out sideways and lean backwards, thus risking a loss of balance. Both manoeuvres are hazardous.

For the purposes of argument each vertical height zone can be divided into three parts, as shown in Fig. 8. Lifting actions performed at more than about half arm's length can only be regarded as acceptable if the weight is low. Lifting actions at more than arm's length will require the trunk to be inclined forwards and therefore should be avoided altogether, unless the weight is **very low**.

	Men			Women		
	Short	Ave	Tall	Short	Ave	Tall
Height	165	177	188	153	164	174
Shoulder height	134	145	156	124	134	143
Elbow height	103	112	121	96	103	111
Knuckle height	72	78	85	69	75	81
Knee height	52	57	62	48	53	57
Arm length	64	69	74	58	63	68

Source: Pheasant (1986, 1991)

FIG. 8 contd.

All dimensions in cm.

THE LOAD

What is a safe load? This question has no easy answer. At the very least it will depend upon the circumstances. A person whose back is in a vulnerable state may be at risk when handling loads which would be well within the safe capacity of a normally fit person. Unfortunately, the warning signs of an impending attack of back pain are not always apparent – either to the individual concerned or to anybody else. In practice, therefore, it will be difficult or impossible to guard against this sort of risk.

In many respects, the best guide as to whether a particular load should be regarded as too heavy to handle, is the sensation of effort entailed for the individual concerned. If a load feels too heavy, then it probably is too heavy. Similarly, if you find that a particular lifting or carrying task makes you feel unduly fatigued or out of breath, then this is a good indication that it is beyond your capacity.

In general a **bulky** load will tend to be both **more difficult** and **more hazardous** to handle than a **compact** load of the same weight. The centre of gravity of the bulky load will be further from the lifter's body, so it will have a greater leverage about the fulcrum of the spine, and will also be more likely to put the lifter out of balance. Wide and long loads may pose particular handling problems; as may loads which are unstable or difficult to grip. The level of risk involved in handling a particular load will also depend upon factors such as obstructions in the working area which limit foot placement, the height range of the lift, and so on.

For a number of reasons, therefore, it is genuinely difficult to be specific about the weight of load which is acceptable in a given situation. But very often this is the wrong way of looking at the problem. Instead, you should be asking whether the working system as a whole is ergonomically satisfactory; that is, does it conform to what is generally regarded as good practice in methods of manual handling?

However, there clearly does come a point at which a load is too heavy, given the nature of the situation in which you are handling it. The guidelines given in the following section may be a useful starting point in considering these questions. But it must be stressed that they are intended as a rough guide only, and in practice it is necessary to evaluate each situation on its own merits. The bottom line is that **there is no such thing as a safe load.**

In practice, the tasks which are most difficult to assess are often the ones which involve the frequent handling of relatively light loads. Although each individual effort may be harmless in itself, the cumulative effect of repeated bending, twisting or lifting actions may be considerable, particularly if they are combined with a high static workload.

GUIDELINES FOR ASSESSMENT: LOAD WEIGHT

The following guidelines are based on the HSE Manual Handling Guidance on Regulations (1992), and are similar to figure 8 of the present text (see pp 20-21). Rather than having a verbal description of each vertical and horizontal lifting zone, however; it shows **guideline weights** in kilograms.

These guideline weights are shown in Table 1. They are considered to define a boundary, beyond which the risk of injury is sufficiently great to warrant a more detailed assessment of the system of work. It is important however, that even where manual handling tasks fall within these limits, they should still be eliminated or improved where it is reasonably practicable to do so; and it should be noted that the limits may be exceeded *where a more detailed assessment shows that it is safe to do so, having regard always to the employer's duty to avoid or reduce risk of injury, where this is reasonably practicable.*

Table 1: **Guideline Weights**

Height Range	Less than half arm's length Kg	Between half arm's length and full arm's length Kg
Shoulder height – full height	10	5
Elbow height – shoulder height	20	10
Knuckle height – elbow height	25	15
Mid lower leg – knuckle height	20	10
Below mid lower leg	10	5

Source: Health and Safety Executive (1992) p.43

The guideline weights given in Table 1 are for lifts performed less than once per minute, under relatively favourable conditions – a compact, stable load which is easy to grasp, with an upright non-twisted trunk, unobstructed workspace, satisfactory environmental conditions and so on. Under these circumstances, the guideline figures are held *to give reasonable protection to nearly all men and between one half and two thirds of women. To provide the same degree of protection to nearly all working women, the guideline figures should be reduced by about one third.* It is also noted that *even for a minority of fit, well-trained individuals working under favourable conditions, any operations which would exceed the guidelines figures by more than a factor of about two should come under very close scrutiny.*

The present authors take this to mean that where the guideline figure is exceeded by a factor of more than about two, the lifting action is likely to be unacceptably hazardous.

It may be useful to think of the guideline figures as a benchmark defining a notional boundary of risk. This benchmark may need to be shifted downwards for some people – for example, the less able half of the female working population, elderly workers and so on. At a level of loading equivalent to about twice the guideline figure is another benchmark, beyond which the level of risk might be considered unacceptably high. Between the upper and lower benchmarks lies a region in which a steadily increasing number of people are exposed to a steadily increasing degree of risk. (This is the present authors' interpretation of the matter.)

GUIDELINES FOR ASSESSMENT: TWISITING AND FREQUENCY OF HANDLING

The HSE Manual Handling: Guidance on Regulations (1992) also suggests that the guideline weights should be reduced, if the lift involves twisting or is more frequent. It provides correction factors for both of these circumstances. These are summarised in Table 2.

Table 2: **Correction Factors for Twisting and Frequency of Handling**

Reduce the guideline weights by the percentages shown		
Twisting	45% ○	10% ○
	90%	20%

	1-2	30%
Frequency of handling (per minute)	5-8	50%
	more than 12	80%

Source: Health and Safety Executive (1992) p. 44

Table 3: **Correction Factors for Stooping**

Reduce the guideline weights by the percentage shown		
	20°	25%
Stooping	45°	35%
	90°	50%

GUIDELINES FOR ASSESSMENT: STOOPING

The HSC Consulative Document (1991) also suggested that the guideline weights should be reduced, if the lift involves stooping. Whilst the correction factors shown in Table 3 were not included in the final HSE Guidance on Regulations (1992), the present authors consider that they are important and should be considered in any assesment.

GUIDELINES FOR ASSESSMENT: CARRYING, PUSHING AND PULLING

The HSE Manual Handling: Guidance on Regulations (1992) also suggests that the guideline weights can be applied to carrying. Here it is assumed that the load is held against the body and is carried no further than about 10m without resting. For greater distances, guideline figures may need to be reduced. In respect of pushing and pulling, the guideline figure for starting or stopping the load is suggested as

25kg; whilst for keeping a load in motion, a guideline figure of about 10kg is suggested. For further details on these guidelines and others (eg for handling while seated) see the HSE Guidance on Regulations (1992), pp. 43-45. It is also noted that the load which a team of two or more lifters can handle safely is less than the sum of the individual capacities of the members of the team. For a two person team, the safe capacity is approximately two thirds of the sum of their individual capacities; for a three person team, the safe capacity is approximately half the sum of their25kg; whilst for keeping a load in motion, a guideline figure of about 10kg is suggested. For further details on these guidelines and others (eg for handling while seated) see the HSE Guidance on Regulations (1992), pp. 43-45. It is also noted that the load which a team of two or more lifters can handle safely is less than the sum of the individual capacities of the members of the team. For a two person team, the safe capacity is approximately two thirds of the sum of their individual capacities; for a three person team, the safe capacity is approximately half the sum of theirindividual capacities. If slopes or steps are to be negotiated, the capacity is diminished further.

REST PAUSES

Rest pauses are important for recovery from muscular fatigue. Again it is difficult to be specific but the following rules of thumb are worth bearing in mind:

- frequent short pauses tend to be more beneficial than infrequent long pauses

- the time required for recovery will be less if the individual concerned takes a rest before the sensations of fatigue become pronounced

- it is always a bad idea to work on to the point of exhaustion.

© Stephen Pheasant and David Stubbs

Assessment template: the task, the load, the working environment, the individual, other factors.

This checklist is intended as an aid to the evaluation of working practices. An answer of YES to any of these questions indicates a potential problem area.

THE TASK

MANUAL HANDLING ACTIVITY

1. Does the task require the person to support a load or exert a sustained force for more than a short period whilst:

   (a) lifting?
   (b) lowering?
   (c) carrying?
   (d) pushing?
   (e) pulling?
   (f) other (eg throwing or controlled dropping)?

HANDLING POSTURES

2. Is the handling action performed with the arms extended away from the body?

3. Is the handling action performed outside an acceptable range of height, given the nature of the load? (See page 21.)

   (a) Is it necessary to handle heavy loads outside the preferred range of heights (ie handler's knuckle to elbow height)?
   (b) Is it necessary to handle a load below mid lower leg height?
   (c) Does vertical distance lifted result in awkward movements?

4. Does the handling action require force exertions whilst:

    (a) stooping forward?
    (b) leaning or reaching sideways?
    (c) twisting the body?
    (d) using only one hand?
    (e) sitting?

STATIC LOADING

5. When handling, is it necessary to work for prolonged periods in the same posture, especially if:

    (a) stooping forward?
    (b) crouching?
    (c) the hands are above mid-torso height?
    (d) bending sideways or rotated?
    (e) twisted?

6. Do the task demands prevent the worker from changing position at will?

7. Are workers required to take their weight on one leg?

8. Do heavy loads need to be precisely manoeuvred?

FREQUENCY

9. Are handling tasks frequently repeated?

    (a) Is it necessary to perform more than 12 handling actions per minute?
    (b) Is it necessary to handle heavy loads more than 5-8 times per minute?
    (c) Is it necessary to perform more than 1-2 handling actions per minute? (See page 25.)

10. Is the work machine paced?

DURATION

11. Do individuals work continuously without adequate recovery time?

12. Do individuals perform the same tasks continuously throughout the working day?

13. Do external factors influence the pace of work or the time period for its completion (eg incentive schemes, piece work, 'job and finish')?

TEAMWORK

14. Do workers perform handling activities as members of a team?

15. Are there occasions when assistance may not be available?

16. Could the weight of the load be unevenly distributed between the handlers at any stage of the task?

OVERALL PHYSICAL WORK

17. Does the overall physical workload seem unreasonably heavy, considering the strength and fitness of the workforce?

THE LOAD

18. Does the weight of the load, or its resistance to movement, exceed recommended guidelines? (See page 23.)

19. Is the weight of the load unevenly distributed?

20. Could the contents shift unexpectedly during the handling manoeuvre?

21. Could the handler be unaware of the above factors?

SIZE AND SHAPE

22. Is the object too bulky for the handler?
    When the load is handled does it restrict:

    (a) the handler's vision?
    (b) the handler's movement?

23. Is the load non-uniform in shape?

24. Is the load difficult to grip firmly (eg slippery, greasy, rounded)?

25. Is the person's task made more difficult through the lack of marking or labelling of the load?

CONDITION

26. Is the load:

    (a) hot?
    (b) cold?
    (c) wet?
    (d) dirty?
    (e) contaminated?
    (f) contained in flimsy or flexible packaging?
    (g) animate?

27. Are there sharp edges or projections?

28. Can the fingers be trapped when gripping the load?

29. If the load is damaged or spilt, will the contents be hazardous? (COSHH)

30. Are gloves necessary when handling the load?

THE WORKING ENVIRONMENT

OBSTRUCTIONS

31. Are there obstructions in the working area which prevent the worker from keeping the load close to the body when handling?

    (a) Is it necessary to reach over obstructions?
    (b Is it necessary to reach into containers?
    (c) Is the worker prevented from adopting the most advantageous foot placements?
    (d) Are heavy or frequently used objects stored in inaccessible places?

SLIPS, TRIPS AND FALLS

32. Are slipping, tripping or falling hazards found in the areas where handling occurs?

    (a) Is the floor slippery?
    (b) Are there steps or changes of level?
    (c) Are there things to trip over?

(d) Does the floor need cleaning?

(e) Is there rubbish or clutter which should be removed?

(f) Can the workplace move or sway unexpectedly?

ACCESS AND CLEARANCE

33. Are there problems of access or clearance for the load, for a tall or bulky person, which cause awkward postures or movements during the handling activity? Are there:

(a) headroom limitations?

(b) narrow aisle widths or passageways?

(c) things to bump into?

(d) limitations on legroom under work surfaces (for sitting people)?

(e) limitations on toe recessess under working surfaces (for standing people)?

GENERAL

34. Are there problems with:

(a) lighting levels?

(b) heat?

(c) humidity?

(d) cold?

(e) wind force?

(f) ventilation?

(g) dust?

(h) noise?

THE INDIVIDUAL
AGE

35. Are any workers:

(a) less than 21 years?

(b) older than 55 years?

SUITABILITY FOR HANDLING WORK

36. Do any workers have:

    (a) limited range of motion in limbs and/or back?
    (b) heart or respiratory problems?
    (c) any history of hernias?
    (d) any musculoskeletal disorder, especially a previous history of back pain?
    (e) any temporary impairment or debility?

37. Are any workers pregnant?

38. Does any worker have specific difficulties in carrying out the manual handling tasks allotted to him/her?

KNOWLEDGE AND TRAINING

39. Could the risks of the handling activity be reduced further if workers had clearer understanding of:

    (a how potentially hazardous loads may be recognised?
    (b) how to deal with unfamiliar loads?
    (c) the proper use of handling aids?
    (d) the proper use of personal protective equipment?
    (e) features of the working environment that contribute to safety?
    (f) the importance of good housekeeping?
    (g) factors affecting individual capability?
    (h) the basics of good handling technique?

PROTECTIVE CLOTHING

40. Are there problems with regard to clothing or personal equipment?

    (a) Does the clothing hamper or constrain the worker's movements?
    (b) Are there items of safety clothing which are – required but not readily available; readily available but not appropriate; or both readily available and appropriate but not used:

gloves?

boots?

headgear?

eye protection?

other?

OTHER FACTORS

41. Is there anything else which makes the task more difficult or hazardous than it needs to be?

Having analysed and evaluated existing working practices, you are in a position to decide upon the most effective course of action to remedy the problems which they pose.

For example, is it possible to solve the problem:

- by changing the layout of the working area, to allow people to work in a better way?

- by redesigning the load, to make it easier to handle?

- by providing mechanical lifting aids of some kind?

- by allocating more people to the job, to reduce the overall burden on each person?

- by training the workforce in safer working practices?

Alternatively, can the working system be redesigned to eliminate the need for handling the load altogether?

TRAINING

TRAINING COURSES

The content of a typical training course could be divided into three areas:

- **knowledge**

- **procedures and practices**

- **skills**

In practice, these may be mixed up together in various combinations. But the distinctions between these components are worth bearing in mind, because they pose different sorts of training problems. It is also worth distinguishing between safety training as such, and safety propaganda. The former is concerned with the imparting of information and the acquisition of skill; the latter is concerned with persuading people to make use of skills and knowledge they already have and to follow correct working procedures.

A certain amount of background knowledge concerning anatomy, body mechanics, etc helps to put the practical content of a training course into context. The way this is taught needs to be carefully matched to the audience. For example, the requirements of a group of office workers would be different from those of a group of engineers. The knowledge element in a course can be taught in a 'classroom' type of environment, although practical demonstrations are always an advantage. But the procedures and skills of lifting should really be taught in the working environment under realistic working conditions, and using the sorts of loads which will be handled on the job.

The distinction between skills and procedures is often blurred, but it has important consequences nevertheless. An individual may be familiar with the correct procedures for lifting a certain kind of load, but be unskilled in its execution and conversely, may become skilled in unsafe working practices. Failure to comply with correct procedures may sometimes be overcome by persuasion in one form or another, but lack of skill cannot be overcome by these means. Skills are sometimes taught as if they are procedures – 'doing it by numbers'. Some skills can be acquired in this way, at least in the early stages. But the execution of a smoothly coordinated lifting action is a skill which requires practice; and coaching by an experienced trainer who has the ability to identify and correct bad habits. This is no easy matter.

It is sometimes said that we remember:

    10% of what we **read**
    20% of what we **hear**
    30% of what we **see**
    50% of what we **see and hear**
    and
    70% of what we **do for ourselves**

Posters and leaflets may be useful adjuncts to safety training, particularly on a propaganda basis to encourage compliance with procedures. They are, however, no substitute for participative programmes of learning by doing, involving discussions of practical problems and 'hands on' exercises in the working situation.

The training session can thus become a collaborative exercise in problem solving in which the trainer learns from the students as well as the other way around, both bringing their own areas of knowledge and expertise to the learning situation. In this way, the trainer can gain valuable insights into current working practices which can be carried forward into subsequent ergonomic improvements.

DRESSING FOR WORK

Students should be advised to attend the training session wearing old, loosely fitting clothing which will not hamper their movements. Women in particular should be reminded to wear sensible shoes and not to wear short or tight skirts. Tracksuits or boiler suits are probably best of all.

THE BASIC LIFT

The lift shown in Fig. 9 is generally considered to be the foundation of good lifting technique, although in practice its applications are limited.

The basic lift should be practised initially using a box-like load which is not more than about 30 cm square and which is heavy enough to involve some sensation of

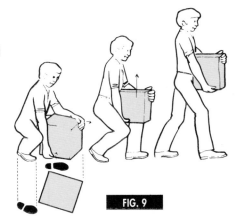

FIG. 9

effort, but not so heavy as to tire the lifter if it is lifted twenty or thirty times during a practice session. Around 5 kg is probably about right for most people. In the first instance, the load should be lifted from the floor on to a low bench or table. As an aid to learning, the lift can be taught in the following stages, but the overall aim should be to achieve a well coordinated, easy and natural pattern of movement, rather than attempting to follow a self-conscious lifting drill which has been learned by rote.

1. **Foot placement:** Start with the load between the feet. The leading foot should be in line with the side of the box, pointing in the direction of movement, with the toes level with the front edge of the box.

2. **Knees bent/back straight:** Get down to the level of the load by bending the knees and hips. Tuck the chin in, and keep the back straight 'from head to tail'. Lean forward a little to get over the load, but do not incline the trunk more than is absolutely necessary. Avoid putting one knee on the floor – this makes for an unstable lifting action. Deep knee bends may also be a problem. They can place an excessive strain on the knee joints and on the thigh muscles which straighten the leg. People with knee problems or weak thigh muscles may find it difficult to lift correctly for this reason.

3. **Grip:** It is important to get a full, firm, secure grip on the load. Loads which are frequently handled should be designed with this in mind. Grip the box at the upper outer corner on the side of the leading foot, tilt it slightly and grip the opposite corner with the other hand. Other hand placements may be better in some cases, depending on what is to be done with the load.

4. **Lift:** Move the load by leaning forward over it a little, keeping the rear arm straight. Pull the box firmly into contact with the body, moving the rear hand forward along the lower edge of the box. Stand up in one coordinated movement, keeping the load in contact with the body throughout.

5. **Lowering:** To lower the load, reverse the procedure, bending the hips and knees whilst tilting the load to avoid trapping the fingers.

Varying the Load

When the trainees have mastered the basic lifting actions on a compact and easily handled load, they can then start to experiment with more difficult loads. For this purpose, it may be useful to have a range of boxes of up to 60 cm square and weighing up to 25 kg. **Each individual trainee must learn to recognise the limits of their strength and lifting capacity, so as to avoid those situations in which they may be at risk of overexertion.** The remainder of the training course should be based upon those type of loads which the trainee is likely to encounter in their everyday work. Procedures for lifting a number of commonly encountered 'difficult loads' are described below.

Using Body Weight

Many lifting instructions talk about 'using body weight' to move the load. This is said to 'take the effort out of work'. Earlier it was noted that body weight must be used as a counterbalance when lifting outside the footbase. But the idea that body weight can be used to actually lift a load is somewhat confusing. It is sometimes possible, however, to move a load horizontally by using its own momentum, having first got it moving by using the body's own momentum. Having done so, it may be possible to swing the load upwards with relatively little effort. Tricks like this take practice and they can only be usefully employed on relatively light loads.

- Above all, lift the load smoothly – don't be a jerk!

The Ergonomic Approach

The ergonomic approach to safe lifting is applicable both to the design of working procedures which will be performed on a regular basis and to the minimisation of risk in the performance of 'one off' manual handling tasks. In the latter case, trainees must learn to plan their own working activities according to good ergonomic principles. For example:

- is the working area clear and free from obstructions?

- can the load be modified in some way to make it easier to lift?

- can the load be turned around so that the 'heavy side' (ie the centre of gravity) is close to the body?

- can the lift be carried through to completion without interruption?

- would it help to use a trestle or platform as a halfway stage?

- how many people are required to safely lift the load?

- would it be better to put the load on a trolley or in a wheelbarrow, or to use some other kind of mechanical aid?

In general:

- STOP, THINK, LIFT

TEAMWORK

The lifting of loads by two or more people presents its own particular set of risks. In general these risks will be minimised if the members of the team are well matched for height and if one person acts as 'team leader', using a predetermined set of commands such as 'ready, steady, lift' etc.

In team lifting it is also important that the people concerned should have sufficient space to manoeuvre as a group, sufficient handholds on the load and so on. This may necessitate putting the load on a stretcher, sling or similar.

HANDLING SACKS

The preferred method for sack handling will depend on its size, weight and carrying distance. Light sacks (less than about 20 kg) may be carried for short distances on the shoulder or clasped in front of the body. For heavier sacks or longer distances a sack trolley is preferable. In applying the following lifting procedures, remember what has previously been said about 'safe loads'.

(i) **Lifting from the floor** (Fig. 10)

The underlying principles are the same as those previously described for the basic lift. Stand at the end of the sack that is easiest to grip. Take up the starting position for the basic lift; grasp the end of the sack, and leaning forward, set it upright. Now reposition the feet and change grip. One hand clasps the sack against the body and the other is placed below it. To raise the sack on to the shoulder, a lifting platform can be used as an intermediate stage. This allows the hands and feet to be repositioned and gives a more comfortable starting position for the second part of the lift. Reposition the feet and change the grip. Set the sack upright and bend the knees and hips to get it on to the shoulder.

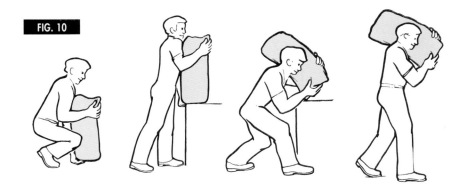

FIG. 10

(ii) **Lifting and carrying from a platform or lorry** (Fig. 11)

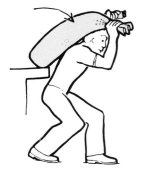

The sack is held at the top, the knees are bent and the sack tilted forward to take the weight. Then in one smooth movement straighten the legs and move off.

(iii) **Carrying sacks on the shoulders**

If not too heavy, a sack can be carried on one shoulder. But the bulkier it is, or the longer the carrying distance, the more tiring it will be for the neck, shoulder and arm muscles. People who habitually carry loads on their shoulders are liable to suffer from neck problems, which is a good argument for using a sack trolley or some other form of transport.

FIG. 11

When carrying on the shoulder, it is best to start from a platform. Stand with the back to the platform, ease the sack on to the shoulder, bending the knees before taking the weight. The sequence for lowering is the reverse of lifting. Lower the sack from the shoulder to the platform, or if safe to do so, ease it off the shoulder and drop it. If the sack has to be lowered under control, bend the hips and knees, and slide it back off the shoulders.

(iv) **Two person lift** (Fig. 12)

The principles are again similar to those of the basic lift. Two people stand on either side of the sack, which is first set upright. The outer foot is the leading foot and points in the direction of movement. The leading hand takes the upper corner of the sack. Be sure that only one of the pair gives the word of command. To obtain a better grip, especially for big sacks, a strong wooden or metal bar, slightly longer than the width of the sack, may be placed underneath it.

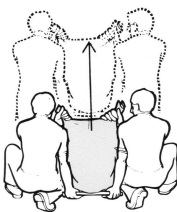

FIG. 12

Long Loads

Long loads present special handling problems. They are less easy to control than compact loads and weight for weight they therefore pose a greater level of risk. Particular problems may arise with long loads which can bend in the middle, such as carpets or thin planks of wood.

(i) **One person lift** (Fig. 13)

The stages of this procedure are similar to those described for sacks. First use the basic lift technique to up-end the load. Then lift it on to the platform, keeping it in a vertical position, as close as possible to the body. Raise the load to the shoulder by bending the knees until the shoulder is level with the point of balance of the load. Then carry the load horizontally balanced on the shoulder. Alternatively, carry the load by hugging it to the chest.

If the load is too long or too heavy to handle in this way, get help. If no help is available, it may be possible to raise one end of the load and drag it along the ground.

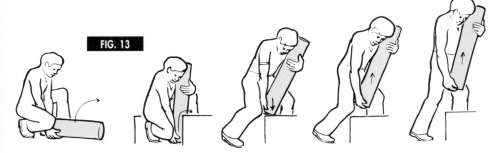

FIG. 13

(ii) **Two person and Team lifting** (Fig. 14)

Two people lifting a long load should start at the heavy end. Using the basic lift technique they raise the load in two stages: firstly to hip height; then, having changed grip to shoulder height, one person supports this end of the load on her shoulder. The other person goes to the opposite (lighter) end and lifts it on to his shoulder in two stages, using a platform. As in all team lifting, good timing is essential.

Some long loads need to be carried in teams of more than two. Ideally, the members of these teams should be as similar in height as possible. Alternatively, the tallest person should be at one end, with the others spaced at suitable distances along the load. Or the load can be handled using slings, with the team members in pairs along its length. The sling passes over the opposite shoulder and is held in both hands. But when loads are this difficult, it is generally better to transport them on a trolley, or some other kind of wheeled conveyance.

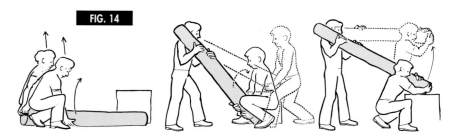

FIG. 14

DRUMS AND BARRELS

Drums and barrels present particular hazards and should not be handled by the uninitiated. Some can weigh over 250 kg and once on the move they are a menace to life, limb and property. Because of this, no advice is offered here except to urge caution and the need to find alternative safer systems of work.

SHEET MATERIAL (Fig. 15)

Single-handed lifting and carrying of sheet material is an inherently hazardous activity. It necessarily involves twisting; and when outdoors, a strong wind can cause the load to act like a sail. The safest, and usually the quickest, way is for two people

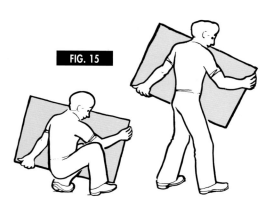

FIG. 15

to handle the sheet. If only one person is available, the sheet should not be longer than their arm span. Tip the sheet up on to one corner, grasp it safely and lift it, keeping the head and back as straight as possible. Sheet materials which have dangerous or fragile corners should be protected. (This is particularly important for glass.) Gloves and carrying tools should be used.

PUSHING AND PULLING (Fig. 16)

The strength of a pushing or pulling action depends on foot placement and on the conditions underfoot. Some research findings seem to indicate that, for a given amount of horizontal force, pushing results in a higher level of spinal loading than pulling. Pushing actions can also fix the rib cage, making breathing more difficult. All else being equal, pulling is, therefore, probably preferable to pushing, although pushing will obviously be safer if there is a possibility of the load getting out of control. Loads on wheels may be a problem on slopes – it is safer to be above the load rather than below it. The best way of shifting a heavy load on the flat is to put your back against it and push it, using the strong muscles of the legs and thighs – but the problem with this method, of course, is that you cannot see where you are going.

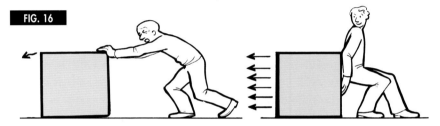

FIG. 16

CARRYING

Carrying involves static muscle loading. Carrying tasks may therefore lead to the rapid onset of muscular fatigue involving the back, shoulder, arm or hand muscles – depending on how the load is supported. Weight for weight, a load carried on the back or shoulders results in a lower level of spinal loading than one carried in front of the body. And a single heavy load carried in one hand will result in a more rapid onset of fatigue, particularly in the shoulder, arm and hand muscles, than two lighter loads carried one in each hand. The onset of fatigue may be delayed by frequently changing hands. In order to minimise the levels of muscular fatigue which result from carrying loads, the following points are recommended:

- use mechanical aids wherever possible

- keep loads light. If possible divide large and heavy loads up into smaller and lighter ones, even if this means making more return trips

- minimise the distance. A series of short return trips is preferable to one long carrying trip

- take regular and frequent rest breaks

Mechanical Lifting Aids

Having identified potential problem areas using the risk assessment checklist described earlier, tasks may be redesigned or mechanised in order to reduce or eliminate their inherent hazards. One way of doing this is by the provision of lifting aids, such as:

1. Levers can be fitted to the load to increase the mechanical advantage of the lifting action – for oil drums, gas cylinders, manhole covers etc.

2. Handles – such as hooks and slings – can be fitted to the load to make it easier to grip.

3. Wheels – such as sack trolleys, luggage trolleys and wheelbarrows – may be fitted to the load to make it easier to transport.

4. Platforms or trestles may be provided to allow the load to be handled at the most convenient height. These must be stable and structurally capable of bearing the load.

5. Other more complex mechanical aids include: palletisers, fork lift trucks, conveyors, cranes and hoists. These and similar aids can be very effective in reducing the physical hazards of manual handling, but other safety problems can arise if insufficient thought is given to their installation and use. For example, fork lift truck operators require training, and vehicle movements around the shop floor and work areas require careful planning to avoid accidents and injuries to operators and pedestrians alike.

   Similarly, conveyors must be guarded against mechanical entrapment, and maintenance considerations of systems, especially space and access, are essential to ensure safe and continuous operation. Conveyor speed must also be considered, as this will dictate the pace of the work, whether loading or unloading.

In selecting either a simple or a more complex aid to lifting and handling, consider the following questions. Does it:

- reduce the level of hazard?

- reduce the level of physical stress?

- create a new hazard?

- meet the approval of the workforce?

- operate over the full range of conditions where its use is planned?

- prolong the time taken to complete the operation?

- accommodate the gloved hand?

- require training in its use?

- offer the potential for abuse?

These are some of the issues that should be discussed as part of the participative approach to devising safer working systems for lifting and handling loads.

FURTHER INFORMATION

OFFICIAL PUBLICATIONS

Council of Ministers of the European Community (1991).

Council Directive on the Minimum Health and Safety Requirements for the Manual Handling of Loads where there is a Risk, Particularly of Back Injury to Workers. Fourth Individual Directive within the meaning of Article 16 (1) of Directive 89/39/EEC, 90/269/EEC, Official Journal of the European Communities 21.6.90, No L 156/9-13, Brussels.

Health and Safety Commission (1991). *Manual Handling of Loads. Proposals for Regulations and Guidance.* Consultative Document CD36, Health and Safety Executive, London.

Health and Safety Executive. *Manual Handling: Manual Handling Operations Regulations, 1992* Guidance on Regulations, Health and Safety Executive, London

BOOKS

Buckle, P (1987). *Musculoskeletal Disorders at Work.* Taylor and Francis, London.

Pheasant, ST (1986). *Bodyspace – Anthropometry, Ergonomics and Design.* Taylor and Francis, London.

Pheasant, ST (1991). *Ergonomics, Work and Health.* Macmillan, London.

Troup, JDG and Edwards, FC (1985). *Manual Handling and Lifting. An Information and Literature Review with Special Reference to the Back.* Health and Safety Executive, London.

HSE Manual Handling: *Solutions You Can Handle* (1994), Health and Safety Executive, London.

Troup, Lloyd, et al. (1992) *The Guide to the Handling of Patients.* NBPA, Middx.

INDEX

INDEX